Wall Pilates Workout

Maximize Your Workout with Wall Pilates: Strengthen, Tone, and Energize Your Body

David Loxley

TABLE OF CONTENTS

INTRODUCTION

Welcome to the world of Pilates! It's unlikely that if you're reading this book, you already know about Pilates and all of its benefits for your body and mind. Pilates is a low-impact workout method that stresses deliberate movement and breathing to enhance balance, flexibility, strength, and posture. Physical therapists, chiropractors, and other healthcare professionals frequently recommend it as a popular type of exercise for people of all ages and fitness levels due to its rehabilitative benefits.

In this book, we'll be focusing specifically on wall Pilates, a variation of Pilates that uses the wall as a prop to enhance and intensify your Pilates workouts. Adding a new depth to your Pilates routine, pushing your body in new directions, and improving your fitness are all possible with wall Pilates. Wall Pilates is a fun, efficient, and accessible approach to get fit and healthy, regardless of whether you are an experienced Pilates practitioner or a novice seeking to try something new.

So what is wall Pilates precisely, and how is it different from regular Pilates? A wall is used as a prop in the Pilates exercise program known as "wall Pilates" to offer stability, resistance, and support. You can add a new dimension to your Pilates exercises and increase the difficulty and intensity of your movements by using the wall as a prop. Pilates wall exercises involves pressing against, leaning against, or using the wall as a support or anchor to challenge your body in new ways.

The fact that wall Pilates is so adaptable and can be used by people of different ages and fitness levels is one of its biggest advantages. Wall Pilates can help you reach your objectives whether you're healing from an injury, trying to strengthen your core, or just want to mix up your Pilates routine. Wall Pilates can also benefit individuals with balance concerns or those who might feel unsteady during classic Pilates movements by offering a solid platform and support.

We'll cover the fundamental Pilates postures and principles, the advantages of wall Pilates, and a variety of wall Pilates exercises that concentrate on various body parts.

Prior to getting started with the workouts and exercises, it's critical to understand that wall Pilates is not a replacement for medical guidance or treatment. We strongly advise speaking with your healthcare provider before beginning any new fitness program if you have any medical ailments or fears, or if you're not sure if wall Pilates is right for you.

Also, when performing wall Pilates exercises, it's important to pay attention to your body and move at your own pace. It's vital to begin carefully and gradually increase the intensity and length of your workouts, just like with any other sort of exercise. Avoid overextending yourself or attempting exercises that are above your current capacity for fitness or ability.

With those important considerations in mind, we invite you to explore the world of wall Pilates and discover the many benefits and possibilities it offers. Wall Pilates is an excellent approach to achieving your fitness objectives and advance your Pilates practice, whether you want to increase your flexibility, tone your muscles, strengthen your core, or just enjoy a fun and challenging type of exercise.

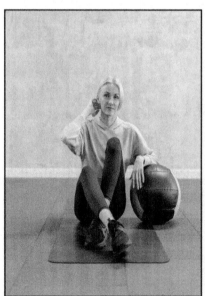 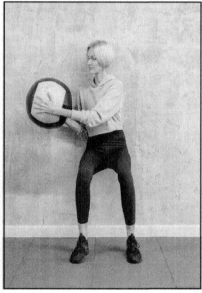

CHAPTER ONE

HISTORY OF PILATES

The Pilates method was established in the early 20th century by German-born physical trainer Joseph Pilates. In the beginning, Pilates was known as "Contrology" and Joseph's own experiences and observations of physical fitness and rehabilitation techniques had an impact on the creation of the discipline.

Joseph Pilates was born in 1883 in Monchengladbach, Germany. He had rickets, rheumatic illness, and asthma as a child, which sparked an early interest in physical fitness and health. He practiced gymnastics, yoga, and martial arts in addition to working as a performer and boxer. He created a set of exercises to aid in the rehabilitation of wounded soldiers while serving as a nurse in internment camps during World War I.

After the war, Joseph settled in New York City and started instructing dancers and other athletes in the Pilates method. His approach was founded on the concepts of breath work, regulated movements, and mind-body integration. He emphasized how crucial it was to build a solid core, or "powerhouse," as he saw this as the basis for both fitness and good health.

The original Pilates exercises, which were done on a mat, emphasized building strength, flexibility, and control. Joseph, however, also created a number of specialized tools to improve and amplify the Pilates exercises. The Cadillac, the Reformer, the Wunda Chair, and the Magic Circle were a few of these equipment. These tools helped the Pilates exercises by offering resistance, stability, and additional difficulties.

During the 1940s and 1950s, Pilates became more popular in the US, especially with actors and dancers. Yet, it wasn't until *Romana Kryzanowska,* a pupil of Joseph Pilates, opened the first Pilates studio in New York City in the 1990s that Pilates gained widespread popularity. Today, Pilates is a well-liked form of exercise for people of various ages and fitness levels and is done all over the world.

At the age of 84, Joseph Pilates passed away in 1967. But his influence continues thanks to the numerous pupils and teachers who carry on his methodology. Along with this evolution, the Pilates method has undergone numerous adjustments and adaptations to accommodate diverse body types and fitness levels. There are many distinct types of Pilates practice available today, including classical, contemporary, and fusion Pilates, which integrates Pilates with other kinds of exercise like yoga or barre.

PRINCIPLES OF PILATES

Six guiding principles serve as the cornerstone of the exercises and serve as the basis for the Pilates method. These principles are concentration, control, centering, precision, breath, and flow. Pilates practitioners can achieve a greater degree of involvement, focus, and physical progress by comprehending and putting these principles into practice.

Pilates demands a great degree of mental attention and concentration. Practitioners must concentrate on each movement, each muscle, and each breath while being totally in the present. To develop a mind-body link that improves awareness, control, and accuracy is the goal.

Control
Control is the foundation of Pilates. The exercises are carried out with intentional, exact movements that employ the muscles in a controlled, conscious manner. Avoiding momentum and jerky movements in favor of smooth, fluid movement that promotes maximum engagement and efficacy is the goal.

Centering
The core of Pilates is the body's center, or its "powerhouse." This is a reference to the muscles that support and stabilize the body, specifically those in the lower back, hips, and buttocks. To support their motions and correct their posture, practitioners are taught to engage and strengthen these muscles.

Precision

In Pilates, precision is key. Each action is carried out in a precise manner with attention to every detail and the right alignment. Its accuracy guarantees that the exercises are efficient, secure, and healthy for the body.

Breath

Breathing is an important factor of Pilates and is utilized to help with movement, calm the body, and improve attention. Practitioners are instructed to breathe deeply and diaphragmatically to revitalize their muscles and oxygenate their bodies.

Flow

Finally, Pilates emphasizes the importance of flow, or the smooth and continuous movement from one exercise to the next. This flow keeps the body constantly engaged and aids in maintaining the mind-body connection.

Pilates practitioners can increase their strength, flexibility, balance, posture, and overall physical health by putting these principles into practice. Another benefit of Pilates is its capacity to lower stress levels, improve mental clarity, and foster relaxation and overall wellbeing.

It's worth noting that the Pilates method is not the only one that uses these ideas. The value of focus, control, centering, precision, breath, and flow is also emphasized in many other types of exercise, including yoga, martial arts, and dance. Yet, the Pilates method differs from other kinds of exercise due to its distinctive approach, techniques, and equipment.

BASIC PILATES POSITIONS AND MOVEMENT

Pilates is a popular form of exercise that has gained a reputation for its focus on strength, flexibility, and mental clarity. The motions and positions used throughout the practice are intended to stretch and strengthen the muscles, increase flexibility and balance, and encourage relaxation and well-being. We will examine some of the fundamental Pilates poses and motions that serve as the basis for this distinctive and powerful exercise regimen in this article.

The Hundred

The Hundred is one of the most iconic Pilates exercises and is often used as a warm-up exercise. Start by lying on your back with your knees bent and your feet flat on the floor to do the Hundred. Straighten your arms in front of you and lift your head, neck, and shoulders off the floor. Start breathing quickly and briefly while pumping your arms up and down. Aim for a count of 100.

The Roll-Up

The Roll-Up is a classic Pilates exercise that targets the core muscles. Lay on your back, knees straight, and arms extended above your head to complete the roll-up. Roll up one vertebra at a time, lifting your head, shoulders, and body slowly until you are sitting. Using your core muscles the entire time, slowly return to the beginning posture.

The Single Leg Circle

The Single Leg Circle is an exercise that targets the hips and lower body. Lay on your back with your legs straight up in the air to execute this workout. Start circling the opposite leg in a clockwise way while keeping one leg straight and stable, then switch to a counterclockwise motion.

The Swan

The Swan is an exercise that targets the upper back, shoulders, and chest. Lay on your stomach and position your hands just below your shoulders to do the Swan. Lifting your chest off the floor while keeping your elbows close to your sides, extend your arms in front of you. For a few breaths, hold this position before lowering yourself back down.

The Plank

The Plank is an exercise that targets the core muscles and helps to improve overall stability and balance. Start in a push-up position with your arms straight and your hands shoulder-width apart to complete the plank. Keep your hips level and your shoulders directly above your hands while engaging your core muscles and holding your body in a straight line.

The Side Plank

The Side Plank is a variation of the Plank that targets the obliques and side muscles. Start in a typical plank position, then shift your weight to one hand and lift your opposing arm straight up into the air to complete a side plank. After a few breaths, maintain this posture before shifting to the opposite side.

The Bridge

The Bridge is an exercise that targets the glutes and lower back. Lie on your back with your knees bent and your feet flat on the floor to execute the Bridge. Squeezing your glutes and using your core muscles to lift your hips upward and toward the ceiling. For a few breaths, hold this position before lowering yourself back down.

The Teaser

The Teaser is an advanced Pilates exercise that targets the core muscles and requires a high level of strength and control. To perform the Teaser, sit on the ground with your legs extended straight out in front of you. Lift your legs and torso off the ground as you start to roll backward, and extend your arms straight in front of you. Before rolling back down, pause for a few breaths in this position.

IMPORTANCE OF BREATH

Breathing is an essential function of the human body, and it is something that we often take for granted. Nevertheless, our physical, mental, and emotional health can all be significantly impacted by how we breathe. The breath is regarded as the basis of the practice in several wellness disciplines, including Pilates, yoga, and meditation. We shall discuss the significance of breathing and how it contributes to general health and wellbeing in this article.

The breath is first and foremost a vital component of our physical wellbeing. The oxygen the body needs to function correctly is delivered to it through breathing. The synthesis of energy, control of metabolism, and body detoxification all depend on oxygen. We can expand our lung capacity, take in more oxygen, and improve circulation when we breathe deeply and deliberately. This can result in more energy, a stronger immune system, and greater physical health in general.

Conscious breathing has a huge effect on our mental and emotional health in addition to its positive effects on our physical health. Since breathing and the nervous system are closely related, controlling our breathing can help us feel more at ease and relaxed. The parasympathetic nerve system, which is in charge of the "rest and digest" response, can be stimulated by slow, deep breathing.

As a result, emotions of relaxation and well-being may be enhanced while stress, anxiety, and tension are reduced.

The breath is also a potent instrument for self-awareness and mindfulness. We become more in the present moment and are better able to tune into our thoughts, emotions, and physical sensations when we focus on our breath. This can enhance our ability to control our thoughts and emotions and help us become more self-aware. Even in the midst of confusion or tension, we can build an inner sense of serenity and tranquility by concentrating on our breath.

Furthermore, in practices like Pilates, breath is a fundamental component of the practice itself. Breath is used in Pilates to encourage appropriate form and alignment, engage the core muscles, and enable movement. During difficult exercises, the breath is used to support and steady the body as well as to encourage a sensation of flow and ease in the action. In this way, the breath becomes an essential component of the practice and aids in fostering increased awareness and control of the body and mind.

Our physical, mental, and emotional wellbeing are all directly impacted by our breath. We may improve our general well-being, foster better physical health, and lessen stress and anxiety by developing a conscious and aware relationship with our breath. Breath is a crucial component of exercises like Pilates because it facilitates improved mobility, increased awareness, and a closer relationship with our bodies. We may tap into the power of the breath and promote a stronger sense of balance, harmony, and vitality by integrating mindful breathing into our daily life.

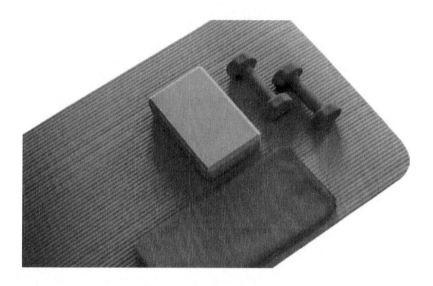

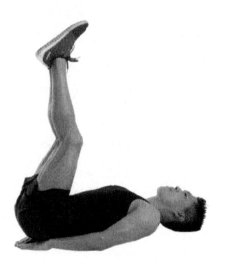

CHAPTER TWO

THE WALL AS A PROP

In Pilates, a prop is any object that can be used to support, challenge or enhance the exercises. Although a mat is sufficient for many Pilates exercises, a variety of props can be used to add variation, difficulty, and depth to the practice. The wall is one such accessory that can be used to support and improve a number of Pilates routines.

The wall is a flexible prop that may be used for exercises while seated or standing. For novices or anyone wishing to improve their technique, the wall can be used as a support to help with alignment and balance. The wall can be used to add resistance or support during specific motions during some workouts, which will make them more difficult.

The wall can be utilized in standing exercises to help with stability and balance. For instance, during the single-leg stance exercise, the wall can be used as a support to assist the person in maintaining good posture and using their core muscles while balancing on one leg. The pelvic clock exercise, in which the person stands with their back against the wall and rotates their pelvis in a circular motion, can also be done against a wall, can help to relieve stress in the lower back and hips.

The wall can be used as a support for the spine during seated workouts, assisting in maintaining good alignment and enhancing posture. The spine stretch forward exercise can be performed against a wall by sitting with the back against the wall and extending the spine straight front. For people with restricted mobility or back problems, the wall serves as resistance and aids in maintaining the spine's appropriate alignment.

Also, you can use the wall as resistance when performing other exercises. For instance, during the leg pull front exercise, the person stands facing the wall and uses the resistance provided by the wall to contract their core muscles and keep their body stable. The wall can also be utilized for the shoulder bridge exercise, in which the person lies on their back with their feet up against the wall and contracts their glute and hamstring muscles in response to the resistance of the wall.

Overall, the wall is a versatile and useful prop in Pilates, offering support, resistance, and balance during a variety of exercises. It may be utilized in a variety of ways to improve the Pilates experience and is a great tool for both new and experienced practitioners. The wall is a useful component to any Pilates practice, whether it is utilized to offer support and stability or to boost the difficulty of an exercise.

BENEFITS OF USING THE WALL

A variety of benefits come from using the wall as a Pilates prop, such as better alignment and balance, more difficulty, and increased awareness of the body's actions. The benefits of using the wall in Pilates exercises are as follows:

Improved Alignment and Balance

The wall provides a stable surface to support the body during exercises, which can help to improve alignment and balance. The person can check their alignment and make sure they are keeping the right posture and form by using the wall as a reference point for their body. This might be particularly helpful for Pilates newbies who are just getting started.

Increased Difficulty

You can utilize the wall to make some exercises more difficult. With the leg pull front exercise, employing the wall as resistance helps to engage the core muscles and stabilize the body while performing the activity. Strength, flexibility, and endurance can all be improved with the addition of this challenge.

Enhanced Body Awareness

Using the wall in Pilates can help to enhance awareness of the body's movements. People can become more conscious of their alignment, posture, and muscle engagement by using the wall as a reference point. This raised awareness can aid in enhancing general movement quality and reducing injury risk.

Versatility

You can perform standing and seated exercises using the wall as a prop. It can be used to help with balance and stability during standing exercises or to support the spine during seated exercises. The wall is a useful tool for any Pilates practice because of its adaptability, which enables a wide variety of exercises to be performed with it.

Accessible

The wall is a readily available prop that can be found in most homes or Pilates studios. Because of this, it becomes a useful tool for people who might not have access to other equipment like the Cadillac or the Pilates reformer. For individuals who might not want to spend money on pricey equipment, the wall is also an affordable solution.

Relieve of Pain and Discomfort

The back, hips, and legs can all be made more comfortable by using the wall. For instance, the pelvic clock exercise, in which the person rotates their pelvis in a circular motion while standing with their back against the wall, can aid in easing tension in the lower back and hips.

Pilates exercises that involve the wall have a number of advantages, such as better alignment and balance, more difficulty, improved body awareness, adaptability, accessibility, and pain and discomfort treatment. Whether you are a novice or an experienced Pilates practitioner, the wall is a useful prop for your practice and can improve your overall Pilates experience.

HOW TO SET-UP FOR A WALL PILATES WORKOUT

A wall Pilates workout's setup is a quick and easy process that only requires a few simple steps. Here is how to get ready for a Pilates session on the wall:

Find a suitable wall: Look for a clear, flat wall that is free of obstructions and has enough space for you to move around. The wall must be strong enough to bear your weight.

Clear the area: Move any furniture or objects that may be in the way, and clear a space in front of the wall.

Prepare your mat: Lay out your mat in front of the wall, leaving enough space to move around comfortably.

Position yourself: Stand facing the wall with your feet hip-width apart, and your hands at your sides.

Engage your core: Engage your core muscles by pulling your navel towards your spine. Your lower back will be supported and kept in good alignment as a result.

Place your hands on the wall: Reach your arms forward and place your hands on the wall at shoulder height, with your fingers spread wide. Your palms should be facing the wall.

Adjust your stance: Walk your feet back until your arms are straight and your body is at a slight angle. Your feet should be parallel to one another and spaced at hip width.

Check your alignment: Ensure that your shoulders are relaxed and spaced apart from your ears, and that your head, neck, and spine are all in a straight line.

Begin your workout: You are now prepared to start your Pilates session against a wall. As your strength and flexibility increase, progress from easy exercises to more difficult ones.

Here are some guidelines for preparing for a wall Pilates workout:

- If you have limited mobility or balance issues, you can start with the wall at a higher level and gradually lower it as you improve.

- When placing your hands on the wall, be careful to keep your wrists straight and your fingers spread widely. By doing this, you can avoid injuries and distribute your weight appropriately.
- Throughout the workout, pay attention to maintaining perfect alignment and using your core muscles. By doing this, you can increase the exercises' beneficial effects and lower your risk of damage.
- Stop the workout right away and speak with a certified Pilates teacher or medical professional if you feel any pain or discomfort.

Finding a good wall, prepping the space, laying out your mat, positioning yourself, engaging your core, placing your hands on the wall, changing your stance, assessing your alignment, and starting your workout are the simple steps in setting up for a wall Pilates workout. You may prepare yourself for a secure, beneficial, and pleasurable wall Pilates workout by adhering to these easy measures.

CHAPTER THREE

ESSENTIAL WARM-UP EXERCISES

Wall Leg Swings

Targets:
Hip flexors, glutes, and hamstrings

Modifications:
You can modify this exercise by holding onto a chair or railing for balance and support if needed.

Instructions:
1. Stand facing the wall with your feet hip-distance apart and your hands on the wall for support.

2. Shift your weight to one foot and swing the other leg forward and backward, keeping your knee straight and your foot flexed.

3. Repeat several times on one leg before switching to the other leg.

4. You can also swing your leg side to side to target your inner and outer thighs.

Wall Cat/Cow Stretch

Targets:
The spine, hips, and core muscles

Modifications:
You can modify this exercise by doing it on the floor instead of against the wall, or by using a cushion or towel to support your knees.

Instructions:
1. Stand facing the wall with your feet hip-distance apart and your hands on the wall for support.

2. Begin in a neutral spine position with your back flat and your core engaged.

3. As you inhale, arch your back and lift your head up, allowing your belly to drop towards the ground (Cow Pose).

4. As you exhale, round your spine and tuck your chin to your chest, bringing your belly button towards your spine (Cat Pose).

5. Repeat for several repetitions, focusing on moving smoothly and deeply with each breath.

Arm Circles

Targets:
The shoulders and arms

Modifications:
You can modify this exercise by using lighter or heavier weights, or by doing the exercise with one arm at a time.

Instructions:
1. Stand facing the wall with your feet hip-distance apart and your arms extended out to the sides.

2. Begin making small circles with your arms, gradually increasing the size of the circles as you go.

3. After several repetitions, switch directions and circle your arms in the opposite direction.

4. Repeat for several more repetitions, focusing on keeping your shoulders down and your core engaged.

Trunk Twists

Targets:
Trunk, oblique, and core muscles

Modifications:

For those who may find the exercise challenging, they can modify the exercise by placing a yoga block or a pillow behind their back, which will help support their spine and make it easier to twist.

Instructions:

1. Stand with your back against the wall, and your feet about hip-width apart.

2. Place your hands on your hips, and engage your core muscles.

3. Inhale and twist your torso to the right, exhale and come back to the starting position.

4. Inhale and twist your torso to the left, exhale and come back to the starting position.

5. Repeat for 10-15 repetitions on each side.

Single-Leg Bridges

Targets:

The glutes, hamstrings, and lower back muscles

Modifications:

For those who may find the exercise challenging, they can modify the exercise by keeping both feet on the floor, or using a yoga block or a pillow to support their neck.

Instructions:

1. Lie down on your back with your feet flat on the wall, and your knees bent at a 90-degree angle.

2. Lift your right foot off the wall and straighten your leg towards the ceiling.

3. Engage your glutes and hamstrings to lift your hips off the floor, coming into a bridge position.

4. Hold for 1-2 seconds at the top, then lower your hips back down to the floor.

5. Repeat for 10-15 repetitions on each side.

Wall Angels

Targets:

Upper back and shoulders

Modifications:

You can modify this exercise by standing with your back slightly away from the wall, or by using a rolled-up towel or cushion to support your lower back.

Instructions:

1. Stand with your back against the wall and your feet hip-distance apart.

2. Raise your arms up to shoulder height and bend your elbows to make a "W" shape.

3. Slowly slide your arms up the wall, keeping your elbows and wrists in contact with the wall, until your arms are extended overhead.

4. Then, slowly slide your arms back down to the starting position.

5. Repeat for several repetitions, focusing on keeping your core engaged and your shoulder blades down and back.

Wall Push-Ups

Targets:

The chest, shoulders, and triceps muscles

Modifications:

For those who may find the exercise challenging, they can modify the exercise by stepping further away from the wall to decrease the resistance.

Instructions:

1. Stand facing the wall with your hands on the wall at shoulder height, slightly wider than shoulder-width apart.

2. Step your feet back and engage your core muscles, coming into a plank position.

3. Inhale and bend your elbows, lowering your chest towards the wall.

4. Exhale and push yourself back up to the starting position.

5. Repeat for 10-15 repetitions.

Calf Raises

Targets:

Calves and ankles

Modifications:

You can modify this exercise by holding onto a chair or railing for balance and support, or by performing the exercise with one leg at a time.

Instructions:

1. Stand facing the wall with your feet hip-distance apart.

2. Place your hands on the wall for support.

3. Lift your heels off the ground, rising up onto the balls of your feet.

4. Hold for a few seconds, then lower your heels back down to the ground.

5. Repeat for several repetitions, focusing on keeping your core engaged and your feet and ankles in a neutral position.

Shoulder Blade Squeeze

Targets:

The rhomboids and trapezius muscles

Modifications:

For those who may find the exercise challenging, they can modify the exercise by using a smaller range of motion or doing the exercise with the hands at chest level instead of overhead.

Instructions:

1. Stand with your back against the wall, with your feet hip-width apart.

2. Bring your arms up and overhead, with your hands resting against the wall.

3. Inhale and squeeze your shoulder blades together, bringing your elbows towards your sides.

4. Exhale and release back to the starting position.

5. Repeat for 10-15 repetitions.

Wall Sit with Alternating Heel Taps

Targets:
The glutes, quadriceps, and hamstrings

Modifications:
For those who may find the exercise challenging, they can modify the exercise by decreasing the depth of the wall sit, or by keeping both feet on the floor instead of tapping the heel.

Instructions:
1. Stand with your back against the wall, with your feet hip-width apart.

2. Slowly slide your back down the wall, bending your knees and lowering your body into a seated position.

3. Lift your left heel off the ground and tap it against the wall.

4. Return your left foot to the ground and lift your right heel to tap against the wall.

5. Alternate tapping your heels for 10-15 repetitions on each side.

Knee Lifts

Targets:
The lower abdominal muscles

Modifications:
For those who may find the exercise challenging, they can modify the exercise by decreasing the range of motion or by placing their hands on the wall for support.

Instructions:
1. Stand with your back against the wall, with your feet hip-width apart.

2. Bring your hands behind your head, and engage your core muscles.

3. Lift your right knee towards your chest, bringing your elbow towards your knee.

4. Lower your right leg back to the starting position and repeat on the left side.

5. Alternate lifting your knees for 10-15 repetitions on each side.

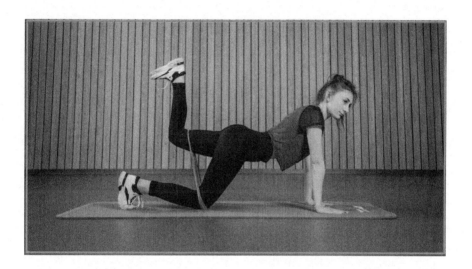

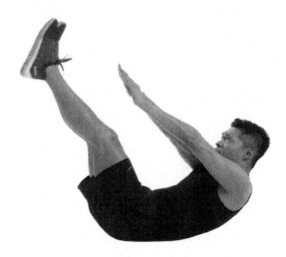

CHAPTER FOUR

CORE WALL PILATES EXERCISES

Wall Pike

Targets:
The abs and lower back

Modifications:
If you're new to wall pikes, start by doing a few repetitions of the exercise while keeping your legs bent. As you get more comfortable with the movement, gradually straighten your legs to increase the difficulty.

Instructions:
1. Stand facing the wall with your feet hip-width apart and your palms flat on the ground in front of you.

2. Walk your feet back until your body is in a straight line and your hips are in line with your shoulders.

3. Engage your core and lift your hips up towards the ceiling, bringing your feet closer to the wall.

4. Slowly lower your hips back down to the starting position, keeping your core engaged throughout the movement.

5. Repeat for the desired number of repetitions.

Wall Plank

Targets:
Abs, Lower back, and shoulders

Modifications:
If you're new to wall planks, start by holding the position for a few seconds and gradually work your way up to longer holds as you get stronger. To increase the difficulty of the exercise, try lifting one leg off the ground or bringing your knees up to your chest.

Instructions:
1. Stand facing the wall with your feet hip-width apart and your hands flat on the wall.

2. Walk your feet back until your body is in a straight line and your arms are straight.

3. Engage your core and hold the position for the desired amount of time.

4. Slowly lower your body back down to the starting position.

Wall Mountain Climber

Targets:
Abs, shoulders and hip flexors

Modifications:

If you're new to wall mountain climbers, start by doing the exercise at a slower pace to get comfortable with the movement. To increase the difficulty, try lifting your hips up towards the ceiling as you bring your knee up to your chest, or try doing the exercise with a resistance band around your ankles.

Instructions:

1. Stand facing the wall with your hands flat on the wall and your feet hip-width apart.

2. Lift one leg off the ground and bring your knee up towards your chest.

3. Quickly switch legs, bringing the opposite knee up towards your chest and lowering the other leg back down.

4. Continue to switch legs as quickly as possible for the desired number of repetitions.

Wall Bird Dog

Targets:

Core, upper and lower back muscles

Modifications:

To decrease difficulty of the exercise, keep both arms and both legs on the wall and lift one arm and the opposite leg at a time. To increase difficulty, extend the lifted leg fully instead of keeping it bent.

Instructions:

1. Stand facing the wall with your hands on the wall at shoulder height.

2. Step back a few feet so that your body forms a diagonal line from your hands to your feet.

3. Lift your right arm and left leg off the wall while keeping your back straight.

4. Hold this position for a few seconds, then lower your arm and leg back down.

5. Repeat with the opposite arm and leg.

6. Do 10-12 repetitions on each side.

Wall Leg Raises

Targets:

Core, lower abdominal muscles

Modifications:

To decrease difficulty, keep both feet on the wall and lift one leg at a time. To increase difficulty, add ankle weights.

Instructions:

1. Lie on your back with your legs extended up the wall.

2. Place your hands under your lower back for support.

3. Lower one leg towards the wall, keeping it straight, until it hovers a few inches off the wall.

4. Lift the leg back up to the starting position.

5. Repeat with the other leg.

6. Do 10-12 repetitions on each leg.

Wall Crunches

Targets:

Core, upper abdominal muscles

Modifications:

To decrease difficulty, keep your knees bent and feet flat on the wall. Extend your legs up the wall and hold a medicine ball or weight if you want to increase the difficulty.

Instructions:
1. Lie on your back with your feet on the wall and your knees bent at a 90-degree angle.

2. Place your hands behind your head.

3. Lift your shoulders off the ground, crunching your upper abs towards your knees.

4. Lower your shoulders back down to the ground.

5. Do 10-12 repetitions.

Wall Side Plank

Targets:
Obliques, hips and shoulders

Modifications:
If this exercise is too challenging, you can perform it with your knees bent and one foot in front of the other.

Instructions:
1. Stand perpendicular to the wall with your feet shoulder-width apart.

2. Place your right forearm on the wall with your elbow aligned with your shoulder.

3. Step your feet away from the wall and lift your hips until your body is in a straight line.

4. Engage your core and hold the position for 30-60 seconds.

5. Lower your hips and repeat on the other side.

Wall Windshield Wipers

Targets:
Entire core (rectus abdominis, transverse abdominis, and obliques)

Modifications:
If this exercise is too challenging, you can perform it with your knees bent and your feet flat on the wall.

Instructions:
1. Lie on your back with your legs straight and your feet against the wall.

2. Extend your arms out to the sides for stability.

3. Slowly lower your legs to one side, keeping them straight and in contact with the wall.

4. Pause briefly, then lift your legs back to center and lower them to the other side.

5. Repeat for 10-15 repetitions on each side.

Wall Oblique Twists

Targets:
Oblique Muscles

Modifications:
If this exercise is too challenging, you can perform it with your hands at chest height, or use a softer wall surface.

Instructions:
1. Stand perpendicular to the wall with your feet shoulder-width apart.

2. Extend your arms straight out in front of you and place your hands on the wall.

3. Engage your core and twist your torso to the right, bringing your left elbow toward your right knee.

4. Return to the starting position and twist your torso to the left, bringing your right elbow toward your left knee.

5. Repeat for 10-15 repetitions on each side.

Wall Side-to-Side Hip Drops

Targets:
Obliques, hips, and thighs

Modifications:
If this exercise is too challenging, you can perform it with your foot on the ground, or use a softer wall surface.

Instructions:
1. Stand perpendicular to the wall with your feet shoulder-width apart.

2. Place your hands on the wall for support.

3. Lift your left leg off the ground and bring it out to the side.

4. Keeping your right leg straight, lower your right hip toward the wall.

5. Lift your hip back up and repeat for 10-15 repetitions on each side.

Wall Roll Down

Targets:
Abdominal muscles, back muscles, and hip flexors

Modifications:

For those who have trouble rolling down all the way, they can start with bending their knees slightly and keeping their fingertips on their thighs. As their flexibility improves, they can slowly start to roll down further until their fingertips reach the ground.

Instructions:

1. Stand with your back against the wall and your feet hip-distance apart.

2. Take a deep breath and engage your abdominal muscles.

3. Slowly start to roll down, vertebrae by vertebrae, until your fingertips touch the ground.

4. Pause for a moment and then start to roll back up to the starting position.

5. Repeat the exercise 8-10 times.

Wall Roll Up

Targets:

Lower back muscles and abdominal muscles

Modifications:

For those who find the exercise too challenging, they can start with a partial roll-up and gradually work up to a full roll-up.

Instructions:

1. Sit on the ground with your back against the wall and your legs straight out in front of you.

2. Engage your core muscles and lift your arms up to shoulder height.

3. Slowly start to roll up, lifting your arms overhead, and reaching towards your toes.

4. Hold the position for a moment and then slowly roll back down.

5. Repeat the exercise 8-10 times.

Wall Knee Tuck

Targets:
The core and hip flexors

Modifications:
For those who find the exercise too challenging, they can start by lowering one leg only partway down the wall and gradually work up to a full leg extension.

Instructions:

1. Lie on your back with your legs straight up against the wall.

2. Place your arms by your sides and engage your core muscles.

3. Slowly lower one leg down towards the ground while keeping the other leg straight up against the wall.

4. Hold the position for a moment and then slowly bring the leg back up to the starting position.

5. Repeat with the other leg.

6. Repeat the exercise 8-10 times.

Wall Teaser

Targets:
Abdominal muscles, hip flexors, and inner thighs

Modifications:
For those who find the exercise too challenging, they can start with a partial roll-up and gradually work up to a full roll-up. They can also use a strap or resistance band to assist in lifting the arms overhead.

Instructions:
1. Sit on the ground with your back against the wall and your legs straight out in front of you.

2. Engage your core muscles and lift your arms up to shoulder height.

3. Slowly start to roll up, lifting your arms overhead, and reaching towards your toes.

4. Hold the position for a moment and then slowly roll back down.

5. Repeat the exercise 8-10 times.

Wall Side Teaser

Targets:
Core muscles and adductors

Modifications:
If you have trouble balancing, you can place your left hand on the wall for support. You can also decrease the range of motion by only bending your knee slightly instead of lowering your body all the way to the wall.

Instructions:
1. Stand facing the wall with your feet hip-width apart and your arms extended straight out in front of you.

2. Slowly lift your right leg off the ground and balance on your left foot.

3. Bend your left knee and lower your body toward the wall while simultaneously extending your right leg out to the side.

4. When you reach the wall, touch it with your right hand, then return to the starting position.

5. Repeat the exercise on the other side.

Wall Roll Out

Targets:
The core muscles

Modifications:
Place a Pilates ball or small cushion behind your lower back to provide support and reduce the strain on your spine. Perform the exercise on your knees instead of your feet to reduce the intensity.

Instructions:
1. Stand facing the wall, with your feet hip-width apart and your hands on the wall at shoulder height.

2. Walk your feet back until your body forms a diagonal line, with your hips over your heels.

3. Engage your core and slowly roll your hands up the wall as you simultaneously roll your spine down towards the floor.

4. Keep your arms straight as you roll forward and inhale, and exhale as you roll back up the wall to the starting position.

Wall Single Leg Stretch

Targets:
The abdominal muscles and the hip flexors

Modifications:
Place a folded blanket or cushion under your head and neck for support and to reduce the strain on your neck. Bend your knees and place your feet on the wall to make the exercise easier.

Instructions:
1. Lie on your back with your hips close to the wall, legs extended up the wall.

2. Place your hands on your left ankle and pull your left leg towards your face as you extend your right leg straight up the wall.

3. Inhale as you switch legs, extending the left leg up the wall and pulling the right leg towards your face.

4. Keep your head and shoulders lifted off the ground and your abdominals engaged throughout the exercise.

Wall Double Leg Stretch

Targets:
The abdominal muscles and the hip flexors

Modifications:

Bend your knees and place your feet on the wall to make the exercise easier. Use a strap around the feet to assist in lifting the legs.

Instructions:
1. Lie on your back with your hips close to the wall, legs extended up the wall.

2. Extend your arms straight up towards the ceiling.

3. Inhale and lower your arms and legs towards the wall, keeping your lower back pressed into the mat.

4. Exhale and lift your arms and legs back up towards the ceiling, keeping your head and shoulders lifted off the ground.

Wall Double Leg Circle

Targets:
The core and hips

Modifications:
If this exercise is too challenging, you can modify it by keeping your head and shoulders on the floor instead of lifting them up. You can also make the circles smaller or slower to reduce the difficulty level.

Instructions:
1. Lie on your back with your hips close to the wall and your legs extended straight up the wall.

2. Place your arms out to the sides for support.

3. Engage your core and press your lower back into the floor.

4. Begin to make slow and controlled circles with both legs, moving in a clockwise direction.

5. After 5-10 repetitions, switch directions and circle counterclockwise.

6. Complete 10-20 repetitions in each direction.

Wall Bridge

Targets:
The glutes, hamstrings, and lower back

Modifications:
If you find this exercise too challenging, you can hold the bridge position for a shorter amount of time or reduce the number of repetitions. You can also place a yoga block or pillow between your knees for added support.

Instructions:
1. Lie on your back with your hips close to the wall and your legs extended up the wall.

2. Place your arms by your sides.

3. Press your lower back into the floor and engage your core.

4. Lift your hips off the ground and hold the bridge position for 5-10 seconds.

5. Lower your hips back down to the floor and repeat for 10-15 repetitions.

Wall Hip Lift

Targets:
The glutes, hamstrings, and lower back muscles

Modifications:
For beginners, this exercise can be done with both feet on the floor, and for a greater challenge, one can lift the legs one at a time while keeping the hips lifted.

Instructions:
1. Lie on the floor facing the wall with the legs bent and feet on the wall.

2. Lift the hips off the floor, forming a straight line from the shoulders to the knees.

3. Hold the position for a few seconds, and then lower the hips back to the floor.

Wall Open Leg Rocker

Targets:
The core muscles

Modifications:

One can modify this exercise by holding onto the ankles or the legs instead of the toes to make it more accessible.

Instructions:

1. Lie on the floor facing the wall with the legs straight up on the wall, toes pointing towards the ceiling.

2. Reach the hands towards the toes, and lift the head and shoulders off the floor.

3. Begin to rock back and forth, using the core muscles to control the movement.

Wall Spine Stretch

Targets:

The back muscles and the hamstrings

Modifications:

One can modify this exercise by bending the knees slightly to take pressure off the hamstrings.

Instructions:

1. Sit on the floor facing the wall with the legs straight up the wall, feet flexed.

2. Reach the arms towards the toes, and begin to slowly roll down, one vertebra at a time, towards the floor.

3. Once the back is flat on the floor, slowly roll back up to the starting position.

Wall Jack Knife

Targets:
The abdominals and obliques

Modifications:
One can modify this exercise by starting with the legs bent, or by holding onto the ankles to make it more accessible.

Instructions:
1. Lie on the floor facing the wall with the legs straight up the wall and the toes pointed towards the ceiling.

2. Reach the hands towards the toes, and lift the head and shoulders off the floor.

3. Lift the hips off the floor, bringing the legs towards the wall and forming a "V" shape with the body.

4. Slowly lower the hips back to the floor, and then repeat the movement.

Wall Side Jack Knife

Targets:
The core muscles, hip flexors and the glutes

Modifications:
For beginners, the exercise can be performed with the legs bent and the feet on the floor. As strength improves, the legs can be extended to make the exercise more challenging.

Instructions:
1. Start by lying on your back with your legs extended and your feet against the wall.

2. Place your hands behind your head, keeping your elbows wide.

3. Lift your legs off the floor and bring them up towards the wall, keeping them straight. As you lift your legs, simultaneously lift your shoulders off the floor and bring your elbows towards your knees.

4. Lower your legs and shoulders back down to the starting position and repeat.

Wall Double Leg Kick

Targets:
The lower back muscles, the hamstrings and glutes

Modifications:

For beginners, the exercise can be performed with a smaller range of motion. Additionally, the exercise can be performed with the hands resting on the wall for support.

Instructions:

1. Start by lying face down with your hands behind your back, palms facing up.

2. Place your feet against the wall with your legs straight.

3. Lift both legs off the floor and kick them towards the wall. As you kick your legs, lift your upper body off the floor and extend your arms back.

4. Lower your legs and upper body back down to the starting position and repeat.

Wall Single Leg Kick

Targets:

The glutes and hamstrings, and lower back

Modifications:

For beginners, the exercise can be performed with a smaller range of motion. Additionally, the exercise can be performed with the hands resting on the wall for support.

Instructions:

1. Start by lying face down with your hands behind your back, palms facing up.

2. Place one foot against the wall with your knee bent, and extend the other leg straight behind you.

3. Lift your bent leg off the wall and kick it towards the wall. As you kick your leg, lift your upper body off the floor and extend your arms back.

4. Lower your leg and upper body back down to the starting position and repeat on the other side.

Wall Heel Tap

Targets:
The core muscles (specifically the obliques)

Modifications:
For beginners, the exercise can be performed with the legs bent and the feet on the floor. As strength improves, the exercise can be performed with the legs straight.

Instructions:
1. Start by lying on your back with your legs extended and your feet against the wall.

2. Place your hands behind your head, keeping your elbows wide.

3. Lift your head and shoulders off the floor and bring your left elbow towards your right knee.

4. Lower your head and shoulders back down to the starting position and repeat on the other side.

Wall Corkscrew

Targets:
The core muscles

Modifications:
If you find this exercise too challenging, try keeping your feet on the floor and only lifting your hips slightly.

Instructions:
1. Lie down on your back with your arms extended to the sides.

2. Lift your legs up and place your feet against the wall.

3. Begin to roll your hips to the right, bringing your legs towards the wall.

4. Use your core to lift your hips and roll them over to the left, lowering your legs towards the floor.

5. Return to the starting position and repeat the movement in the opposite direction.

Wall Mermaid

Targets:
The obliques and intercostal muscles

Modifications:
If you find this stretch too difficult, try placing your hand lower on the wall.

Instructions:
1. Stand facing the wall with your left hand on the wall at shoulder height.

2. Step your left foot back and place your right hand on your hip.

3. Lean to the left, feeling the stretch along the right side of your body.

4. Hold for 20-30 seconds and then switch sides and repeat.

Wall Swan

Targets:
The upper back muscles (including the rhomboids and trapezius muscles).

Modifications:
If you find this exercise too challenging, try moving your feet closer to the wall.

Instructions:
1. Stand facing the wall with your hands on the wall at shoulder height and your feet slightly wider than hip-width apart.

2. Keep your arms straight as you lower your body towards the wall, bending at the elbows.

3. Keep your gaze forward and your neck neutral.

4. Push yourself back up to the starting position and repeat.

Wall Dolphin Plank

Targets:
The core muscles, shoulders, and upper back

Modifications:

To make this exercise easier, you can perform it with your knees on the ground. To make it more challenging, you can lift one leg off the ground or hold the plank for longer periods of time.

Instructions:

1. Stand facing the wall, with your feet hip-width apart.

2. Place your forearms on the wall, with your elbows directly under your shoulders.

3. Walk your feet back until your body is in a diagonal line.

4. Engage your core muscles and hold the plank for 30-60 seconds.

5. Release and repeat for 2-3 sets.

Wall Cat Stretch

Targets:

The spine and core muscles

Modifications:

To make this exercise easier, you can perform it on your hands and knees instead of against the wall. To make it more challenging, you can hold each position for longer periods of time.

Instructions:

1. Stand facing the wall, with your feet hip-width apart.

2. Place your hands on the wall at shoulder height, with your fingers pointing upwards.

3. Inhale and arch your back, lifting your tailbone and head towards the ceiling.

4. Exhale and round your back, bringing your chin towards your chest.

5. Repeat for 10-15 repetitions.

Wall Plank with Shoulder Tap

Targets:

The core, shoulder, and arm muscles

Modifications:

To make this exercise easier, you can perform it with your knees on the ground instead of in a full plank position. To make it more challenging, you can increase the number of shoulder taps or hold the plank position for longer periods of time.

Instructions:

1. Stand facing the wall and place your hands on the wall at shoulder height.

2. Walk your feet back until your body is in a plank position.

3. Keep your core muscles engaged and your body in a straight line.

4. Inhale and tap your right hand to your left shoulder.

5. Exhale and return your right hand to the wall.

6. Inhale and tap your left hand to your right shoulder.

7. Exhale and return your left hand to the wall.

8. Repeat for 10-15 repetitions on each side.

Wall Plank with Leg Lift

Targets:
The core muscles, the glutes, quads, and hip flexors

Modifications:
If this exercise is too challenging, you can start by simply holding a wall plank without lifting your leg. To make it more challenging, you can try lifting both legs at the same time or adding ankle weights.

Instructions:

1. Start by standing facing the wall, about an arm's length away.

2. Place your hands on the wall at shoulder height, fingers spread wide for stability.

3. Step your feet back until your body forms a straight line from head to heels, and engage your core.

4. Lift one leg off the ground, keeping it straight and toes pointed.

5. Hold for a few seconds, then lower the leg and repeat on the other side.

6. Repeat for several reps on each side.

Wall Plank with Arm Reach

Targets:
The core muscles, the shoulder and back muscles

Modifications:
If this exercise is too challenging, you can start by simply holding a wall plank without reaching your arm out. To make it more

challenging, you can try reaching with both arms at the same time or adding a push-up.

Instructions:

1. Start by standing facing the wall, about an arm's length away.

2. Place your hands on the wall at shoulder height, fingers spread wide for stability.

3. Step your feet back until your body forms a straight line from head to heels, and engage your core.

4. Reach one arm forward, keeping it straight and parallel to the ground.

5. Hold for a few seconds, then lower the arm and repeat on the other side.

6. Repeat for several reps on each side.

Wall Leg Lifts

Targets:

The lower abs, hip flexors, and quads

Modifications:

If this exercise is too challenging, you can start by simply holding onto the wall and lifting one leg at a time. To make it more challenging, you can try lifting both legs at the same time or adding ankle weights.

Instructions:

1. Stand facing the wall, about an arm's length away.

2. Place your hands on the wall for support.

3. Lift one leg off the ground, keeping it straight and toes pointed.

4. Hold for a few seconds, then lower the leg and repeat on the other side.

5. Repeat for several reps on each side.

Wall Sit-Ups

Targets:

The core muscles

Modifications:

If this exercise is too challenging, you can start by doing regular sit-ups on the ground. To make it more challenging, you can try holding a medicine ball or adding a twist to the movement.

Instructions:
1. Sit on the floor facing the wall, with your feet flat on the wall and knees bent at a 90-degree angle.

2. Place your hands behind your head, elbows pointing out to the sides.

3. Engage your core and slowly roll up to a seated position.

4. Lower back down to the starting position, and repeat for several reps.

Wall-Assisted Spinal Twists

Targets:
The spine, obliques, and hip muscles

Modifications:
If you have limited mobility, you can modify the exercise by doing the twists while seated in a chair or on the floor. You can also try a gentler variation by twisting just the upper body while keeping the lower body stationary.

Instructions:
1. Stand facing the wall, about an arm's length away from it.

2. Place your hands on the wall at shoulder height, shoulder-width apart.

3. Inhale and lengthen your spine, then exhale and twist your torso to the right, bringing your right hand to your left shoulder blade and your left hand to your right hip.

4. Hold the position for a few breaths, then inhale and return to the starting position.

5. Exhale and repeat the twist to the left.

Wall-Assisted Pike

Targets:
The core, shoulders, and hamstrings.

Modifications:
If you have tight hamstrings or limited flexibility, you can modify the exercise by bending your knees slightly or placing your feet on a step stool.

Instructions:
1. Stand facing the wall, about an arm's length away from it.

2. Place your hands on the wall at shoulder height, shoulder-width apart.

3. Walk your feet back until your body is in a straight line from head to heels and your arms are straight.

4. Inhale and lengthen your spine, then exhale and engage your core as you lift your hips toward the ceiling.

5. Hold the position for a few breaths, then inhale and lower your hips back to the starting position.

Wall-Assisted Roll-Ups

Targets:
The abs, hip flexors, and spinal muscles

Modifications:
If you have difficulty with this exercise, you can modify it by placing a rolled-up towel or cushion under your lower back for support.

Instructions:
1. Lie on your back with your feet against the wall and your legs extended up the wall.

2. Extend your arms up toward the ceiling.

3. Inhale and lengthen your spine, then exhale and engage your abs as you lift your head, neck, and shoulders off the ground.

4. Continue to roll up one vertebra at a time, reaching for your toes with your hands.

5. Hold the position for a few breaths, then inhale and reverse the movement to roll back down to the starting position.

Wall-Assisted Roll-Downs

Targets:
The abs, spinal muscles, and hip flexors

Modifications:
If you have limited flexibility, you can modify the exercise by bending your knees slightly or using a cushion or rolled-up towel behind your back for support.

Instructions:
1. Stand facing the wall, about an arm's length away from it.

2. Place your hands on the wall at shoulder height, shoulder-width apart.

3. Inhale and lengthen your spine, then exhale and engage your abs as you begin to roll your spine down one vertebra at a time, tucking your chin into your chest.

4. Continue to roll down until your hands are at waist height.

5. Inhale and hold the position for a few breaths, then exhale and roll back up to the starting position.

Wall-Assisted Teaser

Targets:
The rectus abdominis, obliques, and hip flexors

Modifications:
You can modify the exercise by bending your knees or keeping your arms lower, closer to your body.

Instructions:
1. Begin by sitting on the floor with your back against the wall and your legs extended in front of you.

2. Place your hands on your thighs and engage your core as you lift your legs and torso up into a V-shape.

3. As you reach your arms forward, continue to engage your core and lift your chest towards your legs.

4. Lower back down with control and repeat.

Wall-Assisted Saw

Targets:
The obliques, spinal rotators, and hamstrings

Modifications:
This exercise can be modified by adjusting the distance between the wall and the feet. A greater distance from the wall will make the exercise more challenging, while being closer to the wall will make it easier.

Instructions:
1. Begin by standing facing the wall, with your feet hip-distance apart and about an arm's length away from the wall.

2. Place your hands on the wall, with your palms facing downward and your fingers pointing towards the ceiling.

3. Inhale as you lengthen your spine, and twist to the right, bringing your left hand towards your right foot.

4. Exhale as you rotate back to center, and then inhale as you twist to the left, bringing your right hand towards your left foot.

5. Exhale as you rotate back to center, and then repeat the movement for several repetitions.

CHAPTER FIVE

UPPER BODY WALL PILATES EXERCISES

Wall Chest Lift

Targets:
Chest muscles, shoulders, and triceps

Modifications:
If you have weak upper body strength, you can start by placing your hands higher up on the wall. You can also decrease the range of motion by only bending your elbows slightly instead of lowering your chest all the way to the wall.

Instructions:
1. Stand facing the wall with your hands placed on the wall at shoulder height.

2. Step back a few feet so that your body is at a slight angle.

3. Engage your core and bend your elbows to lower your chest toward the wall.

4. Press into the wall to straighten your arms and return to the starting position.

Wall Push-Up

Targets:
Chest muscles, shoulders, and triceps

Modifications:
If you have weak upper body strength, you can start by placing your hands higher up on the wall. You can also decrease the range of motion by only bending your elbows slightly instead of lowering your chest all the way to the wall.

Instructions:
1. Stand facing the wall with your hands placed on the wall at shoulder height.

2. Step back a few feet so that your body is at a slight angle.

3. Engage your core and bend your elbows to lower your chest toward the wall.

4. Press into the wall to straighten your arms and return to the starting position.

Wall Doorway Stretch

Targets:
The chest and shoulder muscles

Modifications:

If you find this stretch too difficult, try moving your feet further from the wall.

Instructions:

1. Stand facing the wall with your arms at shoulder height and elbows bent at 90 degrees, your forearms resting on the wall.

2. Step one foot forward, keeping your body upright.

3. Slowly lean forward, keeping your forearms on the wall, and feeling the stretch in your chest and shoulders.

4. Hold for 20-30 seconds and then switch legs and repeat.

Wall Swan Prep

Targets:

Upper back, shoulders, and core

Modifications:

This exercise can be modified by standing farther away from the wall to increase the difficulty or closer to the wall to decrease the difficulty.

Instructions:

1. Stand facing the wall with your feet hip-width apart and your palms on the wall at shoulder height.

2. Keeping your arms straight, lift your chest away from the wall while squeezing your shoulder blades together.

3. Hold for 3-5 seconds, then lower back down.

4. Repeat for 8-12 repetitions.

Wall Chest Opener

Targets:
The chest and upper back

Modifications:
This exercise can be modified by standing farther away from the wall to increase the stretch or closer to the wall to decrease the stretch.

Instructions:

1. Stand facing the wall with your feet hip-width apart and your palms on the wall at shoulder height.

2. Lean into the wall, keeping your arms straight and your shoulder blades down and back.

3. Hold for 30-60 seconds, taking deep breaths.

4. Release and repeat as desired.

Wall Chest Fly

Targets:
The chest, shoulders, and upper arms

Modifications:
This exercise can be modified by standing farther away from the wall to increase the difficulty or closer to the wall to decrease the difficulty.

Instructions:
1. Stand facing the wall with your feet hip-width apart and your palms on the wall at shoulder height.

2. Slowly lower your body towards the wall while bending your elbows, keeping your shoulders down and back.

3. Push yourself back to the starting position while keeping your arms straight.

4. Repeat for 8-12 repetitions.

Wall Row

Targets:
The upper back and biceps

Modifications:
This exercise can be modified by standing farther away from the wall to increase the difficulty or closer to the wall to decrease the difficulty.

Instructions:
1. Stand facing the wall with your feet hip-width apart and your arms straight out in front of you, palms on the wall.

2. Bend your elbows and pull your body towards the wall, keeping your shoulder blades down and back.

3. Push yourself back to the starting position while keeping your arms straight.

4. Repeat for 8-12 repetitions.

Wall Pull-Ups

Targets:
Upper back muscles (including the latissimus dorsi, trapezius, and rhomboids)

Modifications:

For those who may find the exercise challenging, they can modify the exercise by using a lower grip on the wall, or by doing the exercise with their feet on the ground to reduce the amount of weight they need to lift.

Instructions:

1. Stand facing the wall, with your feet hip-width apart and your hands on the wall, shoulder-width apart and at chest height.

2. Inhale and engage your shoulder blades by pulling them down and back.

3. Exhale and lift your body towards the wall, using your back and arm muscles to pull yourself up.

4. Inhale and lower your body back down to the starting position.

5. Repeat for 10-15 repetitions.

Wall Biceps Curl

Targets:

The biceps muscles

Modifications:

For those who may find the exercise challenging, they can modify the exercise by using a lighter resistance band or by shortening the range of motion.

Instructions:

1. Stand facing the wall, with your feet hip-width apart and a resistance band securely anchored to the wall at chest height.

2. Grasp the resistance band with an underhand grip, palms facing up.

3. Inhale and engage your core muscles.

4. Exhale and bend your elbows, pulling the resistance band towards your shoulders.

5. Inhale and slowly lower your arms back down to the starting position.

6. Repeat for 10-15 repetitions.

Wall Triceps Extension

Targets:

The triceps muscles

Modifications:

For those who may find the exercise challenging, they can modify the exercise by using a lighter resistance band or by shortening the range of motion.

Instructions:

1. Stand facing away from the wall, with your feet hip-width apart and a resistance band securely anchored to the wall at waist height.

2. Grasp the resistance band with an overhand grip, palms facing down.

3. Inhale and engage your core muscles.

4. Exhale and extend your arms straight back behind you, keeping your elbows close to your sides.

5. Inhale and slowly bend your elbows to return to the starting position.

6. Repeat for 10-15 repetitions.

Wall Shoulder Press

Targets:

Shoulder muscles (deltoid), triceps, and upper back muscles

Modifications:

For those who may find the exercise challenging, they can modify the exercise by using a lighter resistance band or by shortening the range of motion.

Instructions:

1. Stand facing away from the wall, with your feet hip-width apart and a resistance band securely anchored to the wall at chest height.

2. Grasp the resistance band with an overhand grip, palms facing forward.

3. Inhale and engage your core muscles.

4. Exhale and press the resistance band overhead, straightening your arms.

5. Inhale and slowly lower your arms back down to the starting position.

6. Repeat for 10-15 repetitions.

Wall Pullover

Targets:

Upper back, shoulders and chest muscles

Modifications:

For those who may find the exercise challenging, they can modify the exercise by using a lighter resistance band or by shortening the range of motion.

Instructions:

1. Stand facing the wall, with your feet hip-width apart and a resistance band securely anchored to the wall at chest height.

2. Grasp the resistance band with an overhand grip, palms facing down.

3. Inhale and engage your core muscles.

4. Exhale and extend your arms straight out in front of you, keeping your elbows slightly bent.

5. Inhale and slowly reach your arms back and overhead, allowing your shoulder blades to slide down your back.

6. Exhale and return your arms to the starting position.

7. Repeat for 10-15 repetitions.

Wall Reverse Fly

Targets:

Upper back and shoulders muscles

Modifications:

For those who may find the exercise challenging, they can modify the exercise by using a lighter resistance band or by shortening the range of motion.

Instructions:

1. Stand facing away from the wall, with your feet hip-width apart and a resistance band securely anchored to the wall at waist height.

2. Grasp the resistance band with an overhand grip, palms facing down.

3. Inhale and engage your core muscles.

4. Exhale and extend your arms straight out in front of you, keeping your elbows slightly bent.

5. Inhale and slowly draw your shoulder blades together, bringing your arms out to the sides.

6. Exhale and return your arms to the starting position.

7. Repeat for 10-15 repetitions.

Wall Tricep Press

Targets:

The triceps muscles

Modifications:

For those who may find the exercise challenging, they can modify the exercise by using a lighter resistance band or by shortening the range of motion.

Instructions:

1. Stand facing away from the wall, with your feet hip-width apart and a resistance band securely anchored to the wall at waist height.

2. Grasp the resistance band with an overhand grip, palms facing down.

3. Inhale and engage your core muscles.

4. Exhale and extend your arms straight out in front of you, keeping your elbows close to your sides.

5. Inhale and slowly bend your elbows, bringing your hands towards your shoulders.

6. Exhale and press your hands back out to the starting position.

7. Repeat for 10-15 repetitions.

Wall Chest Press

Targets:
The chest muscles, shoulders and upper arms

Modifications:
For those who may find the exercise challenging, they can modify the exercise by using a lighter resistance band or by shortening the range of motion.

Instructions:
1. Stand facing the wall, with your feet hip-width apart and a resistance band securely anchored to the wall at chest height.

2. Grasp the resistance band with an overhand grip, palms facing down.

3. Inhale and engage your core muscles.

4. Exhale and extend your arms straight out in front of you, keeping your elbows slightly bent.

5. Inhale and slowly bring your arms towards your chest, allowing your shoulder blades to slide together.

6. Exhale and press your hands back out to the starting position.

7. Repeat for 10-15 repetitions.

Wall Tricep Stretch

Targets:
The triceps muscles

Modifications:
To make this exercise easier, you can place your hand on a higher part of the wall or use a resistance band for assistance. To make it more challenging, you can deepen the stretch by leaning further into the wall or using a heavier resistance band.

Instructions:
1. Stand facing the wall, with your feet hip-width apart.

2. Place your hands on the wall with your fingers pointing upwards.

3. Slowly walk your feet back until your arms are straight and your body is in a diagonal line.

4. Keeping your elbows close to your ears, slowly lower your body towards the wall.

5. Hold the stretch for 10-15 seconds, then release and repeat on the other side.

Wall-Supported Swimming

Targets:
The upper back, shoulders, and core muscles

Modifications:
To make this exercise easier, you can use lighter weights or reduce the number of repetitions. To make it more challenging, you can use heavier weights or perform the exercise with one arm at a time.

Instructions:
1. Stand facing the wall, with your feet hip-width apart.

2. Hold a pair of light dumbbells with your palms facing in towards each other.

3. Lean forward and rest your forehead on the wall.

4. Lift your arms up and back towards the ceiling, keeping your shoulder blades down and together.

5. Lower your arms back down to the starting position, and repeat for 10-15 repetitions.

Wall Circles

Targets:
The shoulder joint and upper back.

Modifications:

To make this exercise easier, you can use lighter weights or perform the exercise without any weights. To make it more challenging, you can use heavier weights or perform the exercise for longer periods of time.

Instructions:

1. Stand facing the wall, with your feet hip-width apart.

2. Hold a pair of light dumbbells with your arms extended in front of you.

3. Slowly make small circles with your arms, first in one direction, then in the other direction.

4. Keep your core muscles engaged and your shoulder blades down and together.

5. Repeat for 10-15 repetitions in each direction.

Wall Chest Stretch

Targets:

The chest and shoulder muscles

Modifications:

To make this exercise easier, you can perform it without a resistance band or with a lighter resistance band. To make it more challenging, you can use a heavier resistance band or hold each stretch for longer periods of time.

Instructions:

1. Stand facing away from the wall, with your feet hip-width apart.

2. Hold a resistance band with both hands, and bring your arms up to shoulder height.

3. Place the middle of the resistance band behind your back, and hold the ends of the band in front of you.

4. Inhale and stretch your arms out to the sides, feeling the stretch in your chest and shoulders.

5. Exhale and bring your arms back to the starting position.

6. Repeat for 10-15 repetitions.

Wall Cobra

Targets:
The upper back, shoulders, and chest muscles

Modifications:

To make this exercise easier, you can perform it with your feet on the ground instead of against the wall. To make it more challenging, you can hold each position for longer periods of time.

Instructions:

1. Lie face down on the floor with your feet against the wall.

2. Place your hands on the ground at shoulder height, and press up into a cobra pose.

3. Hold the pose for 10-15 seconds, feeling the stretch in your upper back, shoulders, and chest.

4. Lower back down to the starting position, and repeat for 2-3 sets.

Wall Arm Circles

Targets:

The shoulder joint and upper back.

Modifications:

To make this exercise easier, you can perform it without any weights or use lighter weights. To make it more challenging, you can use heavier weights or perform the exercise for longer periods of time.

Instructions:

1. Stand facing the wall, with your feet hip-width apart.

2. Hold a pair of light dumbbells with your arms extended out to the sides.

3. Slowly make small circles with your arms, first in one direction, then in the other direction.

4. Keep your core muscles engaged and your shoulder blades down and together.

5. Repeat for 10-15 repetitions in each direction.

Wall-Supported Chest Press

Targets:
The chest, shoulders, and triceps muscles

Modifications:
To make this exercise easier, you can perform it with lighter weights or no weights at all. To make it more challenging, you can use heavier weights or increase the number of repetitions.

Instructions:

1. Stand facing away from the wall, with your feet hip-width apart.

2. Hold a pair of dumbbells or resistance bands at shoulder height with your palms facing forward.

3. Lean back into the wall, keeping your arms extended and your elbows slightly bent.

4. Inhale and press the weights or bands away from your chest, feeling the contraction in your chest muscles.

5. Exhale and bring the weights or bands back to the starting position.

6. Repeat for 10-15 repetitions.

Wall-Supported Tricep Press

Targets:
The triceps muscles

Modifications:
To make this exercise easier, you can perform it with lighter weights or no weights at all. To make it more challenging, you can use heavier weights or increase the number of repetitions.

Instructions:
1. Stand facing away from the wall, with your feet hip-width apart.

2. Hold a dumbbell or resistance band in one hand and place the back of your hand against the wall.

3. Keep your elbow close to your body, and inhale as you press the weight or band away from the wall.

4. Exhale and bring the weight or band back to the starting position.

5. Repeat for 10-15 repetitions on each side.

Wall-Supported Bicep Curl

Targets:
The biceps muscles

Modifications:
To make this exercise easier, you can perform it with lighter weights or no weights at all. To make it more challenging, you can use heavier weights or increase the number of repetitions.

Instructions:
1. Stand facing the wall, with your feet hip-width apart.

2. Hold a pair of dumbbells or resistance bands with your arms extended down by your sides and your palms facing forward.

3. Lean back into the wall, keeping your elbows close to your body.

4. Inhale and curl the weights or bands up towards your shoulders, feeling the contraction in your biceps muscles.

5. Exhale and slowly lower the weights or bands back to the starting position.

6. Repeat for 10-15 repetitions.

Wall-Assisted Swan Dive

Targets:
The entire posterior chain of the body

Modifications:
This exercise can be modified by adjusting the distance between the wall and the feet. A greater distance from the wall will make the exercise more challenging, while being closer to the wall will make it easier.

Instructions:
1. Begin by standing facing the wall, with your feet hip-distance apart and about an arm's length away from the wall.

2. Place your hands on the wall, with your palms facing downward and your fingers pointing towards the ceiling.

3. Inhale as you press your hands into the wall, lengthening your spine.

4. Exhale as you begin to fold forward, hinging at the hips and keeping your spine long.

5. Continue folding forward until your torso is parallel to the ground, and your arms are extended behind you.

6. Inhale as you lift your arms up towards the ceiling, keeping them parallel to the ground and your palms facing each other.

7. Exhale as you lower your arms back down to the starting position, and slowly roll back up to standing.

Wall-Assisted Spine Stretch

Targets:
The entire spine, the upper, middle, and lower back muscles

Modifications:
This exercise can be modified by adjusting the distance between the wall and the feet. A greater distance from the wall will make

the exercise more challenging, while being closer to the wall will make it easier.

Instructions:

1. Begin by standing facing the wall, with your feet hip-distance apart and about an arm's length away from the wall.

2. Place your hands on the wall, with your palms facing downward and your fingers pointing towards the ceiling.

3. Inhale as you lengthen your spine, and then exhale as you begin to roll down through your spine, bringing your head towards your knees.

4. Inhale as you begin to roll back up, starting from your tailbone and moving through each vertebrae until you reach your head.

5. Exhale as you return to the starting position.

Wall-Assisted Elephant

Targets:

The lower abdominals and hip flexors, as well as the shoulders and upper back

Modifications:

You can modify the exercise by placing your hands on a chair or bench for additional support.

Instructions:

1. Begin by standing facing the wall with your hands on the wall at shoulder height.

2. Walk your feet back until your body is in a diagonal line from your hands to your feet.

3. Engage your core and lift your hips up towards the ceiling as you draw your legs together.

4. Lower back down with control and repeat.

Wall-Assisted Swan

Targets:

The back muscles, the glutes and hamstrings

Modifications:

You can modify the exercise by placing your hands on the wall at a higher or lower level depending on your flexibility and comfort.

Instructions:

1. Begin by standing facing the wall with your hands on the wall at waist height.

2. Walk your feet back until your body is in a diagonal line from your hands to your feet.

3. Engage your core and hinge forward from the hips as you lower your torso towards the floor.

4. Keep your gaze forward and lift your arms up towards the ceiling as you lift your chest towards the wall.

5. Lower back down with control and repeat.

CHAPTER SIX

LOWER BODY WALL PILATES EXERCISES

Wall Leg Circles

Targets:
Hip flexors, glutes, and quadriceps

Modifications:
If you have tight hamstrings, you can place a folded towel or blanket under

Instructions:
1. Lie on your back with your feet up against the wall.

2. Slowly raise your left leg and circle it around, keeping your knee straight and your foot flexed.

3. Reverse the direction of the circle and repeat the exercise on the other leg.

Wall Side Leg Lift

Targets:
The outer thighs and glutes

Modifications:

You can make this exercise easier by performing the leg lift with your hands on the wall for support. You can also reduce the range of motion if you find the exercise difficult.

Instructions:

1. Stand with your right side facing the wall and place your right hand on the wall for support.

2. Lift your left leg out to the side, keeping it straight and maintaining a neutral spine. Don't let your hips drop or twist.

3. Inhale to lower the leg back down, and then exhale to lift it back up.

4. Repeat for several reps before switching sides and repeating the exercise with your left leg.

Wall Single Leg Circle

Targets:

Hip joint, the hips and thighs muscles

Modifications:

Perform the exercise with both legs at the same time to reduce the intensity.

Place a folded blanket or cushion under your head and neck for support and to reduce the strain on your neck.

Instructions:

1. Lie on your back with your hips close to the wall, legs extended up the wall.

2. Place your hands by your sides with your palms facing down.

3. Inhale and lower your left leg down the wall towards the floor.

4. Exhale and circle your left leg up the wall and towards your body, then back down towards the floor.

5. Repeat the circle 5-10 times, then switch legs.

Wall Squat

Targets:
The quadriceps, glutes, and hamstrings

Modifications:
You can modify the exercise by using a lower or higher wall or chair for support, or by holding weights to increase the difficulty.

Instructions:

1. Start by standing with your back against the wall, feet hip-distance apart, and toes pointing forward.

2. Slide your back down the wall until your knees are at a 90-degree angle, with your knees tracking over your toes.

3. Keep your core engaged and your back flat against the wall.

4. Hold the position for as long as possible, then stand back up.

Wall Lunges

Targets:
The quadriceps, glutes, and hamstrings

Modifications:
You can modify the exercise by holding weights to increase the difficulty or by using a higher or lower wall or chair for support.

Instructions:

1. Start by standing facing the wall with your hands on the wall for support.

2. Step your right foot back, keeping your toes pointing forward and your heel lifted.

3. Bend your left knee to a 90-degree angle, keeping your knee tracking over your toes.

4. Straighten your left leg to return to the starting position and repeat on the other side.

Wall Single-Leg Bridge

Targets:
The glutes, hamstrings, quadriceps, and the core

Modifications:
You can modify the exercise by using a higher or lower wall or chair for support, or by holding weights to increase the difficulty.

Instructions:
1. Start by lying on your back with your feet flat against the wall and your knees bent.

2. Lift your right leg and extend it straight up towards the ceiling.

3. Press into your left foot and lift your hips up towards the ceiling, keeping your right leg extended.

4. Lower your hips back down to the floor and repeat on the other side.

Wall Split Squat

Targets:
The quadriceps, glutes, and hamstrings

Modifications:
You can modify the exercise by using a lower or higher wall or chair for support, or by holding weights to increase the difficulty.

Instructions:
1. Start by standing with your back against the wall and your feet hip-distance apart.

2. Take a large step forward with your right foot, keeping your knee tracking over your toes.

3. Bend your left knee to a 90-degree angle and hold the position for as long as possible.

4. Return to the starting position and repeat on the other side.

Wall Hamstring Curl

Targets:
The hamstring, the glutes, and the calves

Modifications:

To make this exercise easier, place a small towel or pillow under your head for support. To make it more challenging, perform the exercise with one leg at a time.

Instructions:

1. Start by lying on your back, with your heels resting against the wall and your arms resting by your sides.

2. Slowly raise your hips off the floor, keeping your feet flat against the wall.

3. Bend your knees and bring your heels towards your glutes, rolling the ball towards your body.

4. Pause for a moment, then slowly straighten your legs to the starting position.

5. Repeat for the desired number of repetitions.

Wall Step-Up

Targets:

The quads, hamstrings, and glutes

Modifications:

To make the exercise easier, use a lower bench or step. To make it more challenging, hold a weight in each hand.

Instructions:

1. Start by standing facing the wall, with your feet shoulder-width apart and your hands resting on the wall for support.

2. Step up onto the bench or step, keeping your weight on the heel of the front foot.

3. Straighten your leg and lift your body up onto the bench or step.

4. Lower yourself back down to the starting position.

5. Repeat with the opposite leg.

Wall Calf Raises

Targets:
The calf muscles

Modifications:
To make the exercise easier, perform the exercise with both feet at the same time, instead of one foot at a time. To make it more challenging, perform the exercise with one foot at a time, or hold a weight in each hand.

Instructions:

1. Start by standing facing the wall, with your feet shoulder-width apart and your hands resting on the wall for support.

2. Slowly rise up onto the balls of your feet, lifting your heels off the ground.

3. Pause for a moment, then slowly lower yourself back down to the starting position.

4. Repeat for the desired number of repetitions.

Wall Glute Bridge

Targets:
The glutes, hamstrings, and lower back.

Modifications:
To make the exercise easier, perform the exercise with your feet closer to your body, or perform the exercise with both feet at the same time, instead of one foot at a time. To make it more challenging, perform the exercise with one foot at a time, or hold a weight in each hand.

Instructions:
1. Start by lying on your back, with your feet flat against the wall and your arms resting by your sides.

2. Slowly raise your hips off the floor, keeping your feet flat against the wall.

3. Pause for a moment, then slowly lower your hips back down to the starting position.

4. Repeat for the desired number of repetitions.

Wall Fire Hydrant

Targets:
The gluteus medius and minimus muscles

Modifications:
For beginners, it may be helpful to perform this exercise without the use of a wall for support or with a smaller range of motion. To increase the challenge, add ankle weights or perform the exercise with a resistance band around your thighs.

Instructions:
1. Stand facing a wall, with your hands resting on the wall for support.

2. Lift your right leg out to the side, keeping your knee bent at a 90-degree angle.

3. Hold the contraction at the top for a few seconds before lowering your leg back down to the ground.

4. Repeat for 10-15 repetitions on each leg, or until fatigue.

Wall Calf Stretch

Targets:
The calf muscles

Modifications:
To increase the stretch, move your foot farther away from the wall or try a single-leg version of the stretch. To decrease the stretch, move your foot closer to the wall.

Instructions:
1. Stand facing a wall, with your hands resting on the wall for support.

2. Step your right foot back, keeping your heel on the ground and your toes pointed straight ahead.

3. Lean into the wall, keeping your back leg straight and your front knee bent, until you feel a stretch in your calf.

4. Hold the stretch for 20-30 seconds before switching sides and repeating.

Wall Leg Press

Targets:
The quadriceps muscles

Modifications:

For beginners, it may be helpful to perform this exercise with a smaller range of motion. To increase the challenge, add weights or perform the exercise with one leg at a time.

Instructions:

1. Stand facing a wall, with your feet hip-width apart and your hands resting on the wall for support.

2. Keeping your back straight, slowly bend your knees and slide down the wall until your thighs are parallel to the ground.

3. Hold the contraction at the bottom for a few seconds before slowly straightening your legs to return to the starting position.

4. Repeat for 10-15 repetitions, or until fatigue.

Wall Heel Abductor

Targets:

The glutes and inner thigh muscles

Modifications:

If you have trouble balancing, you can lightly touch the wall with your fingertips. To make the exercise easier, you can perform it without lifting your heel off the ground.

Instructions:

1. Stand facing the wall with your feet about hip-width apart.

2. Place your hands on the wall at shoulder height and slightly wider than shoulder-width apart.

3. Slowly lift your left heel off the ground and bring your left knee out to the side, keeping your foot flexed.

4. Hold for a few seconds and then lower your foot back down.

5. Repeat on the other side.

Wall Hamstring Stretch

Targets:

The hamstring muscles

Modifications:

If you have tight hamstrings, you can bend your knees slightly to reduce the intensity of the stretch. To deepen the stretch, you can place a strap or towel around the ball of your foot and gently pull your leg towards you.

Instructions:

1. Lie on your back with your buttocks close to the wall and your legs extended up the wall.

2. Scoot your buttocks closer to or away from the wall to find a comfortable position.

3. Slowly slide one leg down the wall while keeping the other leg straight.

4. Hold the stretch for a few seconds and then slowly slide the leg back up.

5. Repeat on the other side.

Wall Bridge

Targets:
The glutes and the lower back muscles

Modifications:
If you have trouble lifting your hips off the ground, you can place a yoga block or rolled-up towel under your hips to provide extra

support. To make the exercise harder, you can add a resistance band around your thighs.

Instructions:

1. Lie on your back with your knees bent and your feet flat on the wall.

2. Place your hands on the ground by your sides.

3. Lift your hips off the ground, squeezing your glutes at the top of the movement.

4. Hold for a few seconds and then slowly lower your hips back down to the ground.

Wall Leg Lifts

Targets:
The lower abdominal muscles, the hip flexors, and the quads

Modifications:
If you have trouble keeping your lower back on the ground, you can place a small pillow or folded towel under your hips for support. To make the exercise harder, you can add ankle weights or a resistance band around your ankles.

Instructions:

1. Lie on your back with your buttocks close to the wall and your legs extended up the wall.

2. Place your hands by your sides.

3. Slowly lower one leg down the wall, keeping the other leg straight.

4. Raise the leg back up and repeat on the other side.

Wall Knee Bends

Targets:
The quadriceps, glutes, hamstrings, and calves

Modifications:
To modify the exercise, one can perform the knee bends with a wider or narrower stance to focus on different parts of the leg muscles. Additionally, using a resistance band or ankle weights can increase the intensity of the exercise.

Instructions:

1. Stand facing the wall with your feet hip-distance apart and your hands resting on the wall at shoulder height.

2. Slowly lower your body down into a squat position by bending your knees and pushing your hips back.

3. Keep your weight on your heels and make sure your knees are not going past your toes.

4. Pause for a second, then slowly rise back up to the starting position.

Wall Scissor Kicks

Targets:
The lower abdominals, hip flexors, and inner thighs

Modifications:
To make the exercise easier, one can perform the scissor kicks with the legs bent or by decreasing the range of motion. To make it harder, one can perform the scissor kicks with ankle weights.

Instructions:
1. Lie on your back with your hips close to the wall and your legs extended up the wall.

2. Place your hands on the floor by your sides for support.

3. Lower one leg towards the floor while keeping the other leg extended up the wall.

4. Alternate the movement by switching legs and continue to scissor your legs up and down.

Wall Heel Drops

Targets:
The calves

Modifications:
To modify the exercise, one can perform the heel drops with a single leg, hold a weight on the top of the foot, or increase the number of repetitions.

Instructions:
1. Stand facing the wall with your hands resting on the wall at shoulder height.

2. Place one foot against the wall, with your toes pointing up.

3. Slowly lift your heel off the ground and press it against the wall.

4. Lower your heel back down towards the ground, then lift it back up again.

5. Repeat for the desired number of repetitions before switching to the other leg.

Wall Toe Taps

Targets:

The quads, hamstrings, and glutes

Modifications:

The exercise can be modified to be less intense by slowing down the tempo or decreasing the range of motion. Alternatively, the exercise can be made more challenging by increasing the speed or adding resistance bands.

Instructions:

1. Stand facing the wall with your hands resting on it at shoulder height.

2. Extend one leg back and tap your toe against the wall.

3. Quickly switch legs and tap the other toe against the wall.

4. Continue alternating legs for the desired number of reps or time.

Wall Jump Squats

Targets:

The quads, hamstrings, and glutes

Modifications:

The exercise can be modified to be less intense by decreasing the range of motion or by eliminating the jump. Alternatively, the exercise can be made more challenging by increasing the speed, height of the jump or adding weights.

Instructions:

1. Stand facing the wall with your feet shoulder-width apart and your hands resting on the wall at shoulder height.

2. Squat down and explode up, jumping as high as you can.

3. Land softly and repeat for the desired number of reps or time.

Wall High Kicks

Targets:
The glutes, hamstrings, and the core

Modifications:
The exercise can be modified to be less intense by slowing down the tempo or decreasing the range of motion. Alternatively, the exercise can be made more challenging by increasing the speed or adding ankle weights.

Instructions:

1. Stand facing the wall with your hands resting on it at shoulder height.

2. Lift one leg straight up, keeping it as straight as possible, and kick it towards the wall.

3. Return your leg to the starting position and repeat with the other leg.

4. Continue alternating legs for the desired number of reps or time.

Wall Side Lunges

Targets:
The inner and outer thighs, the glutes and hamstrings

Modifications:
The exercise can be modified to be less intense by decreasing the range of motion or by eliminating the jump. Alternatively, the exercise can be made more challenging by adding a resistance band or weights.

Instructions:
1. Stand with your right side facing the wall and your hands resting on it at shoulder height.

2. Step your left foot out to the side and bend your left knee, keeping your right leg straight.

3. Push off your left foot and return to the starting position.

4. Repeat on the other side, stepping out with your right foot.

5. Continue alternating sides for the desired number of reps or time.

Wall Dead Bugs

Targets:
The rectus abdominis, the obliques, the hip flexors and the quadriceps

Modifications:
To make this exercise easier, you can reduce the range of motion or perform the movement without straightening your legs. To make it more challenging, you can extend your arms and legs further away from the wall, or add a resistance band around your feet.

Instructions:
1. Lie on your back with your legs bent and your feet flat against the wall, your arms extended straight up towards the ceiling.

2. Exhale and slowly lower your right arm and left leg towards the floor, keeping your lower back flat against the wall.

3. Inhale and return your arm and leg to the starting position.

4. Repeat the movement with the opposite arm and leg, and continue alternating sides.

Wall Marching

Targets:
The abdominal muscles, hip flexors, and leg muscles

Modifications:
To make this exercise easier, you can reduce the range of motion, or perform the movement without fully extending your legs. To make it more challenging, you can add ankle weights or perform the exercise with a resistance band.

Instructions:
1. Lie on your back with your legs straight up against the wall and your arms at your sides.

2. Engage your core and slowly lower one leg towards the floor while keeping the other leg straight up against the wall.

3. Exhale and bring the lowered leg back up to the starting position while simultaneously lowering the opposite leg.

4. Continue alternating legs as if you are marching in place against the wall.

Wall Plie Squats

Targets:
The glutes, hamstrings, and quads

Modifications:
To make this exercise easier, you can reduce the range of motion or use a stability ball to support your back against the wall. To make it more challenging, you can hold a weight or medicine ball in front of your chest.

Instructions:
1. Stand backing the wall with your feet wider than hip-width apart and your toes turned out.

2. Place your hands on the wall for support and engage your core.

3. Bend your knees and lower your body down towards the floor, keeping your back flat against the wall and your knees in line with your toes.

4. Exhale and push through your heels to return to the starting position.

Wall Reverse Lunges

Targets:
The glutes, hamstrings, and quads

Modifications:
To make this exercise easier, you can reduce the range of motion or hold onto the wall for support. To make it more challenging, you can add a weight or perform the exercise on a balance board.

Instructions:
1. Stand facing the wall with your feet hip-width apart and your hands on the wall for support.

2. Step back with one leg and lower your body down towards the floor, bending both knees to a 90-degree angle.

3. Exhale and push through your front heel to return to the starting position.

4. Repeat the movement with the opposite leg, and continue alternating sides.

Wall Clamshells

Targets:
The gluteus medius and minimus

Modifications:

You can make the exercise easier by reducing the number of repetitions or shortening the range of motion. To make it harder, you can use a resistance band around your knees or add ankle weights.

Instructions:

1. Stand with your back against the wall and feet shoulder-width apart.

2. Place a small ball or rolled-up towel between your knees.

3. Slowly lift your top knee while keeping your feet together and your pelvis stable.

4. Pause at the top and lower back down.

5. Repeat for several repetitions on one side before switching to the other side.

Wall Single Leg Deadlifts

Targets:

The hamstrings, glutes, and lower back muscles

Modifications:

You can make the exercise easier by holding onto a chair or countertop for balance. To make it harder, you can hold a weight in one or both hands.

Instructions:

1. Stand with your back against the wall and feet hip-width apart.

2. Shift your weight onto one foot and lift the other leg slightly off the ground.

3. Hinge forward at the hips, extending the lifted leg straight back and reaching your arms down towards the ground.

4. Keep your standing leg slightly bent and your core engaged to maintain balance.

5. Pause at the bottom and then slowly return to the starting position.

6. Repeat for several repetitions on one side before switching to the other side.

Wall Side Step-Ups

Targets:
The glutes, quadriceps, and hip flexors

Modifications:
You can make the exercise easier by stepping up onto a lower surface or using a wall for support. To make it harder, you can add weight or increase the height of the step.

Instructions:
1. Stand facing the wall with one foot on a bench or step and the other foot on the ground.

2. Place your hands on the wall for support.

3. Step up with your back foot, driving your knee towards your chest.

4. Pause at the top and then slowly lower back down.

5. Repeat for several repetitions on one side before switching to the other side.

Wall Donkey Kicks

Targets:
The glutes and hamstrings

Modifications:

You can make the exercise easier by shortening the range of motion or reducing the number of repetitions. To make it harder, you can add ankle weights or perform the exercise with a resistance band around your ankles.

Instructions:

1. Start on all fours with your hands on the wall and your knees hip-width apart.

2. Lift one leg up towards the ceiling, keeping your knee bent at a 90-degree angle.

3. Squeeze your glutes at the top of the movement and then slowly lower back down.

4. Repeat for several repetitions on one side before switching to the other side.

Wall Standing Figure Four Stretch

Targets:

The hips and glutes

Modifications:

For those with tight hips, move farther away from the wall. Another option is to use a block or towel under the foot for support.

Instructions:

1. Stand facing the wall and place one foot on the wall with the knee bent at a 90-degree angle.

2. Slowly lower the hips down towards the ground and move the foot higher up the wall if possible.

3. Hold the stretch for several deep breaths, then release and switch sides

CHAPTER SEVEN

COOL DOWN EXERCISES

Seated Forward Fold

Targets:
The hamstrings, the back, hips, and calves

Modifications:
For those with tight hamstrings or a limited range of motion, sitting on a folded blanket or block can provide support. Another option is to bend the knees slightly or use a strap to help reach the feet.

Instructions:
1. Sit on the floor with the legs extended in front of you.

2. Inhale and lengthen the spine, reaching the crown of the head towards the ceiling.

3. Exhale and fold forward from the hips, reaching towards the toes or shins. Keep the spine long and avoid rounding the back.

4. Hold the stretch for several deep breaths, then release.

Standing Forward Fold

Targets:
The hamstrings, calves, and lower back

Modifications:
For those with tight hamstrings, bend the knees slightly and place the hands on the thighs. Another option is to use a block to bring the ground closer.

Instructions:
1. Stand with the feet hip-width apart and parallel to each other.

2. Inhale and lift the arms overhead.

3. Exhale and hinge forward from the hips, keeping the spine long and reaching towards the ground.

4. Place the hands on the ground, block or hold opposite elbows with the hands.

5. Hold the stretch for several deep breaths, then release.

Extended Leg Stretch

Targets:
The hamstrings, calves, and lower back

Modifications:

For those with tight hamstrings or a limited range of motion, a folded blanket or block can provide support. Another option is to bend the knee slightly or use a strap to help reach the foot.

Instructions:

1. Sit on the ground with one leg extended in front of you and the other knee bent.

2. Inhale and lengthen the spine, reaching the crown of the head towards the ceiling.

3. Exhale and fold forward from the hips, keeping the spine long and reaching towards the toes or shin of the extended leg.

4. Hold the stretch for several deep breaths, then release and switch sides.

Kneeling Hip Flexor Stretch

Targets:

The hip flexors

Modifications:

To modify this stretch, you can place a cushion or folded towel under your back knee to provide extra support. You can also place your hands on the wall in front of you to maintain balance.

Instructions:

1. Begin by kneeling on the floor with your knees hip-width apart and your toes tucked under.

2. Step your right foot forward so that your knee is directly above your ankle.

3. Keep your left knee on the floor and press your hips forward, feeling a stretch in the front of your left hip.

4. Hold the stretch for 30 seconds to one minute, then release and switch sides.

Backward Lunge Stretch

Targets:

The quadriceps, hamstrings, and glutes

Modifications:

If you have difficulty balancing, you can use a wall for support during the stretch. You can also place your hands on your hips to help stabilize your body.

Instructions:

1. Stand up straight with your feet hip-width apart.

2. Step your right foot back, lowering your right knee toward the floor.

3. Keep your left knee directly above your ankle and press your hips forward, feeling a stretch in the front of your right thigh.

4. Hold the stretch for 30 seconds to one minute, then release and switch sides.

Neck Rolls

Targets:
The neck muscles

Modifications:
To modify this exercise, you can perform smaller, gentler neck movements if you experience discomfort or limited mobility in your neck.

Instructions:

1. Begin by standing up straight with your feet hip-width apart.

2. Drop your chin to your chest and slowly roll your head to the right, bringing your right ear toward your right shoulder.

3. Roll your head back to the center and then to the left, bringing your left ear toward your left shoulder.

4. Continue rolling your head in a circular motion, moving slowly and gently.

5. Repeat for several repetitions, then reverse the direction of the circle.

Shoulder Rolls

Targets:
The shoulder muscles

Modifications:
To modify this exercise, you can perform smaller, gentler shoulder movements if you experience discomfort or limited mobility in your shoulders.

Instructions:
1. Begin by standing up straight with your feet hip-width apart.

2. Roll your shoulders forward, up, back, and down in a circular motion.

3. Repeat for several repetitions, then reverse the direction of the circle.

Torso Twists

Targets:
The back, waist, and hips muscles

Modifications:
If you find it challenging to balance in the twisted position, you can perform the exercise with your back against the wall. Place a block or pillow between your legs to make it easier to maintain the position.

Instructions:
1. Stand with your feet shoulder-width apart, and your back facing the wall.

2. Place your hands on the wall at shoulder height.

3. Slowly twist your torso to the right, keeping your hips facing forward.

4. Hold this position for a few seconds, then twist to the left.

5. Repeat the exercise for 10 to 15 repetitions.

Wall Forward Bend

Targets:
The hamstrings, back, and shoulders

Modifications:
If you have tight hamstrings, you can bend your knees slightly to take the pressure off the backs of your legs. You can also use a strap or towel to help you reach your feet.

Instructions:
1. Stand with your back against the wall, and your feet hip-width apart.

2. Slowly bend forward from your hips, keeping your back straight.

3. Reach for your toes, and hold this position for a few seconds.

4. Slowly roll back up to a standing position.

5. Repeat the exercise for 10 to 15 repetitions.

Wall Shoulder Stretch

Targets:
The shoulders, upper back, and chest muscles

Modifications:
If you find it challenging to reach your hands behind your back, you can use a towel or strap to assist you.

Instructions:
1. Stand with your back against the wall, and your feet hip-width apart.

2. Reach behind your back, and interlace your fingers.

3. Slowly lift your arms away from your body, keeping your shoulders relaxed.

4. Hold this position for a few seconds, then release.

5. Repeat the exercise for 10 to 15 repetitions.

Wall Calf Stretch

Targets:
The calves muscles

Modifications:

If you find it challenging to keep your balance, you can hold onto a chair or wall for support.

Instructions:

1. Stand facing the wall, with your hands on the wall at shoulder height.

2. Step back with your left foot, keeping your heel on the ground.

3. Slowly bend your right knee, and lean forward, keeping your left leg straight. Hold this position for a few seconds, then switch sides.

4. Repeat the exercise for 10 to 15 repetitions on each side.

Wall Figure Four Stretch

Targets:

The hips and the glutes

Modifications:

For those who are less flexible, the foot can be placed lower on the wall or on a lower surface such as a chair. To increase the stretch, you can gently push your right knee towards the wall.

Instructions:

1. Stand facing a wall and place your right foot on the wall with your knee bent.

2. Slowly slide your foot down the wall until your knee is at a 90-degree angle.

3. Cross your left ankle over your right knee and gently press your left knee away from your body until you feel a stretch in your left hip.

4. Hold the stretch for 30-60 seconds, then switch sides and repeat.

Wall Final Twist

Targets:
The spine

Modifications:
For those who have tight hips or hamstrings, the legs can be bent slightly. For those with neck or shoulder issues, the head can remain facing forward or be supported with a pillow.

Instructions:

1. Lie down on your back facing a wall and scoot your hips as close to the wall as possible.

2. Place your arms out to the sides at shoulder height.

3. Bring your knees up to your chest and then extend your legs up the wall.

4. Lower your legs to one side of your body, keeping your shoulders on the ground, and turn your head in the opposite direction.

5. Hold the stretch for 30-60 seconds, then switch sides and repeat.

Wall-Supported Forward Fold

Targets:
The hamstrings

Modifications:
For those with tight hamstrings, the knees can be slightly bent or a prop such as a block can be used under the hands.

Instructions:
1. Stand facing a wall and place your hands on the wall at shoulder height.

2. Walk your feet back until your body is at a 90-degree angle to the ground.

3. Keep your legs straight and hinge forward at the hips.

4. Hold the stretch for 30-60 seconds.

Wall Quad Stretch

Targets:
The quadriceps muscles

Modifications:
For those with balance issues, the stretch can be done with the support of a chair or wall. If it is difficult to reach the foot, a strap or towel can be used to help hold onto the foot.

Instructions:
1. Stand facing a wall and place your left hand on the wall for support.

2. Bend your right knee and bring your heel towards your buttocks.

3. Reach back with your right hand and grab your right foot.

4. Gently pull your foot towards your buttocks to deepen the stretch in your quadriceps.

5. Hold the stretch for 30-60 seconds, then switch sides and repeat.

Wall Hamstring Stretch

Targets:
The hamstrings and thighs

Modifications:
To make this stretch easier, you can use a strap or towel to wrap around the foot and gently pull the leg towards your body.

Instructions:
1. Start by lying on your back with your hips close to the wall and your legs extended up the wall.

2. Your feet should be flexed, and your heels pressing into the wall.

3. Slowly walk your hands towards the wall as you slide your heels down towards the floor.

4. Stop when you feel a stretch in your hamstrings and hold the position for 15-30 seconds.

Wall Spine Stretch

Targets:
The spine, hips, and lower back

Modifications:

If you find it difficult to sit on the floor, you can sit on a folded blanket or pillow to elevate your hips.

Instructions:

1. Sit on the floor facing the wall with your legs crossed.

2. Place your hands on the wall, inhale, and lengthen your spine.

3. As you exhale, slowly walk your hands down the wall and lower your forehead towards the floor.

4. Hold the position for 5-10 deep breaths, then slowly walk your hands back up to a seated position.

Wall Knee-To-Chest Stretch

Targets:

The hip flexors, lower back, and glutes

Modifications:

If you find it difficult to reach your knee, you can wrap a towel or strap around your leg and gently pull it towards your chest.

Instructions:

1. Lie on your back facing the wall with your legs extended up the wall.

2. Bend your right knee and place your foot on the wall.

3. Slowly bring your right knee towards your chest as you exhale, using your hands to help guide it.

4. Hold the position for 15-30 seconds and release.

5. Repeat on the other side.

Wall Figure Four Stretch

Targets:
The hips, glutes, and lower back

Modifications:
If you find it difficult to cross your leg over the opposite knee, you can rest your ankle on the opposite knee instead.

Instructions:
1. Lie on your back facing the wall with your legs extended up the wall.

2. Cross your right ankle over your left knee and slide your left foot down the wall.

3. Gently press your right knee away from your body to deepen the stretch.

4. Hold the position for 15-30 seconds and release.

5. Repeat on the other side.

Wall Downward Dog

Targets:
The arms, shoulders, back, hips, and legs

Modifications:
If you find the full pose too challenging, you can modify by walking your hands higher up the wall or by bending your knees slightly. You can also try the exercise with one foot lifted at a time for an extra challenge.

Instructions:
1. To perform this exercise, stand facing a wall with your hands on the wall at shoulder height, fingers spread apart.

2. Step your feet back and walk your hands down the wall until your body forms an inverted "V" shape.

3. Keep your arms straight, your shoulders down, and your neck relaxed. Your feet should be hip-width apart and your heels should be pressing down toward the floor.

4. Hold the pose for several deep breaths, then slowly walk your hands back up the wall to come out of the pose.

Wall Shoulder Opener

Targets:
The shoulders, chest, and upper back

Modifications:
If you find the stretch too intense, you can adjust the height of your hand on the wall or walk your feet closer to the wall. You can also try the stretch with your arm bent at a 90-degree angle.

Instructions:
1. To perform this exercise, stand with your side facing a wall.

2. Place your hand on the wall at shoulder height and walk your feet away from the wall until you feel a stretch in your shoulder and chest.

3. Keep your arm straight and your shoulder down.

4. Hold the stretch for several deep breaths, then switch sides.

Wall Glute Stretch

Targets:
The hips, glutes, and lower back

Modifications:
If you find the stretch too intense, you can adjust the angle of your legs or place a folded blanket or cushion under your hips for support. You can also try the stretch with your foot on the wall at a lower height.

Instructions:
1. To perform this exercise, lie on your back with your hips close to the wall and your feet flat against the wall.

2. Cross your right ankle over your left knee, then slide your left foot down the wall until you feel a stretch in your right hip and glute.

3. Hold the stretch for several deep breaths, then switch sides.

CHAPTER EIGHT

CONCLUSION

Strengthening, toning, and energizing your body with wall Pilates is a unique and effective method. We have looked at a wide range of wall Pilates exercises in this book that work the core, arms, legs, and back, among other body areas. All fitness levels and needs can be accommodated by altering the exercises in this book, from basic stretches to more complex routines.

Review of the Benefits of Wall Pilates

Pilates on a wall has many benefits. It is first and foremost a fantastic way to tone and strengthen your body. You may work your muscles in new and difficult ways by using the wall as a prop, which can help you get greater results faster. Wall Pilates is also a low-impact workout that is gentle on the joints, making it an excellent choice for people who are healing from injuries or who have chronic pain.

Your range of motion and flexibility can both be enhanced with wall Pilates. You can gradually deepen your stretches and improve your flexibility by utilizing the wall to support your body in certain poses. This can help you avoid injuries, enhance your posture, and simplify daily activities.

The capacity of wall Pilates to strengthen your mind-body connection is another benefit. You can focus on the present and feel less stressed and anxious by using the calm, controlled motions and emphasizing appropriate breathing. Your total health, both mentally and physically, may benefit from this.

How to Incorporate Wall Pilates Into Your Regular Routine

It is simple and versatile to incorporate wall Pilates into your daily practice. The workouts in this book can be modified to meet your schedule and fitness level and can be done at home or in a gym.

Setting up a specified period of time each day to perform a few exercises is one approach to include wall Pilates into your schedule. Depending on your schedule and priorities, this could take as little as 10 minutes or as much as an hour. You can progressively increase your strength and flexibility over time by making it a daily practice.

Making use of wall Pilates as a warm-up or cool-down before or after other forms of exercise is another option to include it in your regimen. For instance, you can warm up your muscles and reduce the risk of injury by performing a few wall Pilates movements prior to a run or a weightlifting session. Alternatively, you can stretch out your muscles and avoid discomfort by performing a few wall Pilates exercises after a workout.

Final Thoughts and Encouragement

The bottom line is that wall Pilates is a flexible and effective technique to enhance your physical and mental health. The exercises in this book can help you develop strength, tone your body, and increase your flexibility whether you are new to Pilates or a seasoned master.

Keep in mind that every person's journey is unique and that development takes time. It's important to pay attention to your body's signals and move at your own pace. Don't give up if you find an activity too challenging. There are numerous alterations and adjustments that can increase accessibility.

Lastly, remember to have fun! Wall Pilates is a demanding and satisfying workout, but it's also supposed to be fun. Do new things and discover your body's capabilities without hesitation. Your fitness goals may well be met, and you can feel your best, with commitment, persistence, and practice.

Printed in Great Britain
by Amazon

20713926R10092